How to Avoid Vomiting

P-MAV
Manual

Peterson Method to Avoid Vomiting

By

Douglas Peterson, DDS

Disclaimer

The P-MAV, as described in this manual is intended to be used in the correct circumstances and situations. When performed incorrectly or when it is not intended or in any circumstance where the suppression of vomiting should be avoided, the result could be dangerous, harmful or even life-threatening.

Until you are confident in the use of the P-MAV for a particular situation, consult with your doctor to determine if the suppression of vomiting is in your best interest.

The author of this manual accepts no responsibility for any outcome resulting from the misuse of this method or misdiagnosis of conditions for which this method was intended.

Contents

What is the P-MAV?

. . . and what's so bad about vomiting?

Few things on earth rival the unpleasant feeling of vomiting. Yuck. It's even unpleasant to write about. We've all been through it at some point in our lives and the best word to describe the experience is simply, miserable! No matter how you cut it, when you know it's coming it is impossible to stop the intense, involuntary muscle contractions and retching associated with vomiting. That is. . . Impossible until now.

The Peterson Method to Avoid Vomiting (or P-MAV for short) is a simple technique that is easy to learn. When used properly and under the right circumstances, it can really save you from a lot of the trauma, distress and discomfort associated with vomiting. There are absolutely no prescription medications needed and therefore no adverse side effects or drug interactions. Additionally, when the P-MAV is successful your symptoms will disappear and you will feel almost instant relief from your nausea.

It's all about the saliva. Prior to vomiting, your body begins to heavily salivate and the glands inside your mouth secrete a substance that initiates vomiting. By observing these salivary changes and learning when they occur, you can bypass the vomiting reflex. The P-MAV teaches you how to avoid vomiting by preventing the ingestion of this specific saliva.

The key to the P-MAV is to use it under the right circumstances. There are times when your body will need to expel the contents of your stomach in order to get rid of a foreign substance or toxin. So it is important to distinguish between the times when vomiting is a necessary part of the nausea cycle and when it is simply the end result. Let us explore some of the more common causes of vomiting and determine if the circumstances justify the use of the P-MAV.

Why Do We Vomit?

Ultimately, we vomit in order to expel the contents of our stomach. Vomiting is a defense mechanism which helps get rid of a toxin or poison that is in the gut. It is also a mechanism to expel food when too much as been consumed. That's it. There are no other reasons for vomiting. However, there are many other circumstances which cause people to vomit. Why?

The question is, 'Why do people vomit when they do not need to empty the contents of their stomach?' What kind of physiologic process is happening which causes the body to vomit even when their stomach contents are normal? That is what we are trying to figure out.

To understand the process, let's take a brief look at the nervous system. The nervous system is divided into two groups - the voluntary and the involuntary nervous systems. The voluntary nervous system, as the name suggests, controls voluntary movements of the body. For example, if you touch a hot stove your response is to quickly move away based on the messages of pain through your nervous system. You are consciously aware of what you are doing and you do it.

The involuntary nervous system, also called the autonomic nervous system, controls systems in your body that are working subconsciously - such as your respiration and the beating of your heart. To some degree you can control these things (holding your breath or increasing your heart rate with exercise) but after a while the autonomic system takes over in order to regulate your body back to normal.

When unusual circumstances put excessive stress on the autonomic nervous system, the body and mind have to compensate in unusual ways in order to get back to normal. Chemical messengers in the form of hormones and neurotransmitters are secreted from specific glands in the body in order to help regulate the affected systems. The sympathetic branch of the autonomic nervous system is switched 'on' when the body needs to speed things up and get things moving faster. The parasympathetic branch does the opposite - slowing down systems as needed.

Vomiting most certainly qualifies as an involuntary (or autonomic) response to particular stresses on your system. Neurotransmitters are released and the message given to the stomach is to vomit, pushing all of its contents back up through the esophagus and out the mouth - an entirely involuntary reaction due to the chemicals released in response to stress.

It is understandable why we would vomit when some toxin or poison is ingested but why do we vomit at other times? Well, the bodily systems that react to poisons are programmed to initiate the "fight or flight" response of the sympathetic branch of the autonomic nervous system. It's an emergency 911 call to the brain saying that something drastic needs to be done and it needs to be done immediately!

When other bodily stresses are extreme, the body does not discriminate between the causes of the stress. The autonomic nervous system kicks in and has the capacity to elicit an equally extreme response to the crisis: the emergency 911 call. As a result the same processes drive the system. Chemical neurotransmitters are released triggering a series of involuntary physical responses.

As the body adjusts to this crisis, the adrenal glands supply adrenaline and cortisone. The heart starts to pump harder and breathing becomes more rapid. Blood flow is redirected away from organs that are not vital to the survival of the organism and toward the systems which will be needed for the physical activity to come. The parasympathetic branch of the autonomic nervous system causes the release of excessive saliva from several glands inside the mouth. This was originally thought to be a mechanism to lubricate the esophagus and protect the teeth from the impending acid soon to be released by the stomach.

If the stimulus creating the stress goes away, the system regulates and symptoms slowly diminish. But, if the stress continues to the breaking point, the effect it has on the body is quick and decisive. The nausea cycle begins and the end result is vomiting.

In emergency situations where the autonomic nervous system is overloaded, the body will do everything and anything it needs to survive the crisis. A whole host of changes take place that are beyond our physical control. Even though vomiting might not be the solution for the current problem, vomiting happens along with the many other critical life-saving strategies employed in a system shutdown and reboot. Once the right chemicals are secreted, the rest is on autopilot.

Reasons to Avoid Vomiting

Let's face it. Vomiting is very repulsive. It can be embarrassing. It can be painful. It can certainly be traumatic - especially after surgery. It smells. It is messy. It is difficult to witness as a parent and difficult to control as a child. It leaves you with a sore throat and a bad taste in your mouth. It makes you dehydrated and sometimes malnourished. It's downright disgusting no matter how you look at it. There are many reasons to try to avoid the process of vomiting.

From a dental perspective, frequent and repeated vomiting can have a lasting and irreversible negative effect on your teeth. Stomach acid is so caustic that it can actually erode the outer layer of tooth enamel. When this happens it can affect your ability to properly chew food and ultimately affect your overall health and nutrition.

The Nausea Cycle

nausea - *a feeling of sickness with an inclination to vomit.*

The nausea cycle has a gradual onset that becomes more and more uncomfortable as long as the causative stimulus continues. Some people experience a rapid onset of symptoms while others may experience them much more gradually. Initially, there is an overall feeling of tiredness or malaise that comes over your body. It becomes difficult to focus on small tasks and attempting to perform specific, tactile movements can exacerbate the condition. As it progresses there may be symptoms of vertigo or dizziness followed by a feeling of nausea in the stomach or head. Unpleasant odors, bright lights or certain sounds can also precipitate the nauseous feeling as it peaks.

The final pre-vomit symptom of the nausea cycle is the metallic tasting, thick, ropy saliva that is secreted from the glands inside your mouth. Once this saliva starts flowing it is a definite sign that your body is on the verge of something beyond your control. And sure enough, within seconds, the retching and vomiting begins.

The progression of these symptoms is common for sufferers of sea sickness, motion sickness, pregnancy related morning sickness, illness, migraine headaches and most other 'common causes of vomiting'. The stimuli may be different in each case but the body's physical reaction to these ailments will precipitate the nausea cycle.

Common Causes of Vomiting

Motion Sickness or Sea Sickness

Pregnancy Related Morning Sickness

Anxiety

Illness

Chemotherapy and Radiation Therapy

General Anesthesia and Surgery

Migraine Headaches

Vertigo

Concussion

Hangover/Alcohol*

Food Poisoning*

Other Causes of Vomiting

*these are examples of when using the P-MAV may not be beneficial

Motion Sickness or Sea Sickness

A very large percentage of the human population suffers from some type of motion sickness. It is difficult to understand why some people do while others do not have this affliction. The causes of motion sickness can vary widely but it is still quite unknown how to prevent or cure the symptoms associated with it. There are many devices and drugs on the market that claim to have the answers but nothing is 100% effective.

> *"The inspiration for the P-MAV stems from my life-long battle with sea sickness. I have enjoyed boating and fishing in the ocean for as long as I can remember. However, when the ocean is rough and the waves are rolling I know that I am going to have a problem with motion sickness. The severity of the sickness will vary - depending on the sea conditions. On rare occasions my sea sickness would result in a bout of nausea followed by cycles of vomiting.*
>
> *Interestingly, directly following the vomiting my body and mind would feel completely better as if there was never a problem - until the cycle started up again about 15-20 minutes later.*
>
> *It bothered me that friends of mine could go out fishing in the same conditions and feel perfectly fine with no signs of illness. Not only would my body feel miserable but my sea sickness slowly turned something that I loved to do (fishing) into something that I started to dread and avoid. Taking drugs would sometimes help but the side effects were uncomfortable and unpredictable."*
>
> *~Douglas Peterson DDS*

People who suffer from motion sickness and sea sickness are unable to enjoy the pleasures of boating, fishing, amusement parks and sometimes even simple things like a ride in the car. The P-MAV, although it may not completely solve the problem, may be the answer many people have been searching for.

If you knew how to avoid the unpleasant nature of vomiting in these situations, perhaps these activities would become much more enjoyable again.

Pregnancy Related Morning Sickness

While developing the P-MAV it was clear that the population of people who stood to benefit mostly by its use would be expectant mothers.

Pregnancy is one of the most wonderful experiences a woman will go through in her lifetime. The miracle of life - it is an undeniably magical time. As incredible as it is, pregnancy puts a woman's body through many physical and hormonal changes and this can be quite stressful at times. As a result, a high percentage of pregnant women have early and frequent encounters with the nausea cycle in the form of what is known as morning sickness.

It is quite a shame actually that such an amazing life experience for a young woman can be marred by such an unpleasant side effect like repeated vomiting. The severity of morning sickness varies greatly - incapacitating some women while others may not be affected at all. Wouldn't it be great if there were a way for women to avoid the muscular stresses and foul nature of the vomiting reflex altogether? Can you imagine the potential stress that is put on a fetus' growth and development if the mother is constantly retching and vomiting?

For pregnant women who are inescapably held prisoner by the terrible nature of morning sickness, your salvation may be right here!

Anxiety

Fear and anxiety can have profound psychological and physiologic effects on the body. For certain, people who suffer from severe anxiety have experienced how the autonomic nervous system is able to take control of their bodies. The mind and the gut are very closely related - not so much in function, but in the nerve pathways and chemical receptors.

As anxiety builds it can make you literally sick to your stomach and as it continues to worsen, the nausea cycle will begin. There are many things that can bring on a feeling of anxiety such as studying for a test, speaking in public, meeting someone for the first time, a job interview, conflicts at work, money problems, medication side effects, trauma, abuse, uncontrollable situations, etc. This list can go on and on but it all comes down to one word - stress.

Anxiety is someone experiencing the fear of what 'might' happen. The feelings associated with this fear are often heightened or exaggerated. A stress on your system causes the autopilot to kick in and try to regulate things. Stress causes your heart rate to increase, your body to sweat and your respiration to quicken. The 'fight or flight' response of the sympathetic nervous system is ready for action. The nausea cycle begins.

If you are one of the many people who suffer from anxiety to the point of vomiting, there may be some help for your condition. Read on.

Illness

Have you or your kids ever had the flu or a stomach virus? Often these illnesses result in multiple bouts of nausea, diarrhea and vomiting. Very unpleasant stuff - especially for children. You body is under attack from a virus and your immune system is doing everything it can to recover. Amidst the crisis your autonomic nervous system is under extreme stress trying to maintain equilibrium.

Symptoms of illness are similar to those associated with the nausea cycle. Fever, sweating, chills, fatigue, low appetite, cough, runny nose, head and body aches, etc. are all common symptoms when your body is under a viral attack. At its absolute worst, vomiting occurs. For a brief time after vomiting you get relief from your other symptoms - until the virus starts to win the battle again and the cycle starts all over. Eventually you get better but the vomiting is what most people remember when they think of some of the worst illnesses they have experienced.

Does the vomiting really need to occur? For stomach viruses this question is certainly debatable. If something is in the stomach and your body would benefit in some way to have it removed, then the vomiting should occur. In many cases however, the vomiting is once again an effect of the autonomic nervous system reacting to extreme stress. The nausea cycle begins and vomiting is the end result.

In order to try to avoid the most unpleasant stage of having a virus or other illness, the P-MAV may be helpful to know. Take caution in using the method under the right circumstances and not in situations where the stomach would actually benefit from emptying its contents.

Chemotherapy and Radiation Therapy

Few things in a person's life can rival the unpleasantness of having to go through therapy for the treatment of cancer. Chemotherapy and radiation are designed to eradicate cancer cells but in the process many normal cells and organ systems are negatively affected. The entire immune system can be compromised and these physiologic stresses often result in the nausea cycle.

Nausea and vomiting are very common side effects for people undergoing cancer treatment. In an already extremely difficult time, frequent vomiting can affect a person's quality of life and result in dehydration, weight loss and malnutrition - all of which are critical to avoid while trying to get healthy again.

Because nausea and vomiting are so common during cancer treatment, a host of anti-vomit or antiemetic medications are used to combat these symptoms. They work by suppressing the release of specific neurotransmitters associated with vomiting. Similar to the pharmacology used to prevent motion sickness, these medications are not 100% successful. Sometimes the addition of steroids will increase the effectiveness of the antiemetic in order to match the strength of the chemotherapeutic agents. By introducing more and more chemicals into an already immunocompromised system, the side effects and drug interactions continue to add stress.

If the P-MAV can be utilized in order to remove just one part of the trauma associated with cancer therapy, wouldn't it be worth a try? Removing some or all of the vomiting (thereby eliminating some of the dehydration, weight loss and malnutrition) could be a vital step in the recovery from such conditions.

General Anesthesia and Surgery

General anesthesia is used in a wide variety of surgeries ranging from the removal of wisdom teeth to cancer treatments to organ transplants and everything in-between. Postoperative nausea and vomiting (or PONV) is a side effect that is quite common in people for a period of time following their surgical procedure and/or use of general anesthetic.

In line with some other common causes of nausea, there seems to be a significantly higher prevalence of PONV among females as opposed to males. Other risk factors which may increase susceptibility to PONV, not surprisingly, include a history of migraines and a history of anxiety. It is also worth noting that volatile anesthetics as well as the duration of the anesthesia both increase a person's chance of experiencing PONV.

Under anesthesia the normal function of a person's central nervous system is temporarily altered. Doctors use drugs and medication to change an individual's body chemistry. While unconscious, people undergo traumatic surgeries that would otherwise be impossible to withstand without the use of the anesthesia. Afterward, it is only natural that the body's automatic systems will begin the process of trying get back to normal function. In response, it is common for the autonomic nervous system to cause PONV during this system wide re-boot.

In order to combat the symptoms of nausea, more chemistry is introduced to the system. Side effects and drug interactions may result but in many cases the risks associated with using the medication to control PONV outweigh the potential complications that could arise as a result of repeated bouts of vomiting. After surgery the body is in a very fragile state and any additional trauma in the early healing stages can be catastrophic. Vomiting is a highly traumatic physical event and that is why many precautions are taken to try to avoid it. That is also why it is often acceptable to take significantly powerful anti-emetic drugs despite other risks or side effects.

Think about the effect that repeated vomiting could have on someone who has just undergone open heart surgery or any type of abdominal surgery that involves stitches or staples to keep a surgical incision closed.

Due to some accidents and trauma to the face, there are situations when a surgeon needs to wire a patient's jaw shut after surgery. The jaw may need to be immobilized for a period of time while healing. Can you imagine experiencing nausea or the urge to vomit while having your mouth wired shut?

If there's a chance that the P-MAV can diminish or eliminate the vomiting stage of the nausea cycle, this method could be immensely beneficial to anyone following a traumatic surgery. It could literally be a life saver.

Migraine Headaches

When migraine headaches get extreme, sufferers often experience nausea. Nausea induced by a migraine may or may not culminate in vomiting, but a sizable percentage of migraine sufferers claim their headaches are causing vomiting. A trend in such cases is the report that vomiting makes the migraine pains go away.

It is more common for female migraine sufferers to complain about nausea than males. There are no definite reasons why nausea and vomiting are common symptoms of migraines. In fact, underlying causes of migraines are mostly unknown. The unusual part of the migraine-nausea cycle is the physiological reason for vomiting as a result of having a headache. Why would the body need to expel the stomach contents in order to feel better? It doesn't. Once again, this is another effect caused by the autonomic nervous system under extreme stress..

During vomiting there is intense pressure in the head and neck while the diaphragm muscles contract causing retching and violent heaving of the gut. If you are suffering from a migraine headache, this is absolutely the last thing that you want to have happen. There is some solace in the knowledge that after vomiting, the symptoms of the headache may diminish or disappear. But wouldn't it be so much better if migraine sufferers could get to the point of feeling better without the actual vomiting taking place? The P-MAV may offer some relief in the final stages of the nausea cycle for people suffering from the most miserable kinds of headaches.

Vertigo

Vertigo is a condition associated with dizziness and balance instability. It is thought that the vestibular system of the inner ear is not properly connecting to the brain which causes the nerve centers responsible for balance and body equilibrium to not function properly. Not surprisingly, these are normally a function of the autonomic nervous system. Typically you do not have to consciously think about walking and staying upright without falling over. Your vestibular system takes care of that for you - on autopilot.

Due to trauma, headache, inflammation, illness, disease, chemical imbalance or other cause, some people develop vertigo and their systems can no longer function automatically in a normal capacity. When the nervous system is stressed trying to self correct, it sometimes reaches its threshold limit. The body's reaction to breaching this limit is to release neurotransmitters and begin the nausea cycle. In extreme cases of vertigo, vomiting is the end result followed by a system reboot. Once again this is a trend identified in many of the common causes of vomiting.

People who suffer from regular bouts of vertigo are fully aware how debilitating it can be. It can come over you in an instant and can be very unpredictable. People with extreme cases sometimes do not leave their homes for fear of having episodes in public. By learning the P-MAV these people can feel more confident with the knowledge that they may be able to control one aspect of their illness. If they are able to avoid the vomiting then perhaps they will regain some of the functionality of life that their condition has taken from them.

Concussion

A concussion is a brain injury that may occur after a blow to one's head that causes the brain to move slightly within the skull. This trauma may temporarily disrupt the electrical activity within the brain so that it stops working properly for a short period of time. This disruption often leads to symptoms of concussion which include headache, confusion, loss of memory and nausea which can also lead to vomiting.

Similar to a migraine headache, a concussion can cause excessive stress to the autonomic nervous system as the body tries to cope with the immediate crisis. Nausea and vomiting may result. The P-MAV may help to eliminate the additional bodily stresses associated with vomiting when someone is suffering from the symptoms of a concussion.

Food Poisoning

There are some circumstances when your body will benefit from expelling its stomach contents as quickly as possible. Vomiting is necessary in order to get rid of poison or toxins that have been ingested. Sometimes the nervous system will react to the toxin and cause an automatic response. Common symptoms of food poisoning include diarrhea, sweating, dizziness, abdominal pain, fever and vomiting.

Sometimes your body will not immediately recognize a toxin in time. For these situations there are medications available which will actually induce vomiting by irritating the gastric mucosa in the stomach and activate the chemoreceptor trigger zone in the brain. It is never advisable to induce vomiting this way unless instructed by a qualified physician.

I hope it is obvious, but in case it's not, the P-MAV is not recommended for use in circumstances where the body would benefit from the act of vomiting. By suppressing the vomit response you may be doing more harm than good.

Hangover and Alcohol

Many people, at some point(s) in their lives have experienced the effects of excessive alcohol consumption. Obviously, some more than others and the degree to which alcohol affects some people can be much more (or less) pronounced. This will depend upon how tolerant your body has become to the effects of alcohol after repeated exposure.

Similar to food poisoning, excessive amounts of alcohol will act as a toxin and your body will react to it. When stressed to the breaking point, the nausea cycle will begin and vomiting will be the end result.

Overindulgence in alcohol can be life threatening and it may be important to allow the body to go through its automatic regulation process of evacuation. For this reason it is not advisable to utilize the P-MAV in these particular circumstances.

Other Causes of Vomiting

There are many other ailments which may lead to the nausea cycle and/or cause vomiting. The previously mentioned reasons are among the most common but there may be other causes of vomiting that could benefit from the P-MAV. It is always important to make sure that the circumstances in which you try to avoid vomiting are warranted. You should never avoid vomiting when it would be more beneficial for your body to empty the contents of your stomach. If you are unsure, consult with your physician.

The Common Trend

What happens almost immediately following a bout of vomiting? In most cases the affected person suddenly and miraculously feels significantly better. The nausea cycle is complete and the symptoms disappear. It really is a wonderful thing going from what feels like the brink of despair to almost instantly feeling normal again.

If you have experienced this common trend at the end of the nausea cycle then you may also remember that in many cases the cycle has its way of coming right back around again. That's why it's called a cycle. It's just a matter of time. Sometimes you will begin to feel the initial symptoms of the nausea cycle again in about 15 to 20 minutes. Sometimes it is longer or shorter depending on your individual sensitivity to the stimulus.

If you're lucky, at the end of the nausea cycle your symptoms may disappear for good. Take solace in the fact that they eventually will be gone for good. It depends upon how many cycles your body has in store for you and for how long you subject yourself to the stimuli that caused the cycle to begin with.

With the P-MAV you can teach yourself how to avoid the single most uncomfortable stage within the nausea cycle - the vomiting. You can essentially trick your body into believing that you have completed the nausea cycle without going through the unpleasantness of the final stage. When successful, you will immediately feel the euphoria associated with the elimination of your nausea symptoms. You feel normal again - and it's a wonderful thing. The best part about it is that you did it without vomiting. Although the cycle may repeat itself again, you will feel much more comfortable knowing that the retching, vomiting, abdominal muscle contractions, taste, smell and mess will not be part of the equation any longer!

It's All About the Saliva

In the scientific study of the nervous systems, we identify the chemical substances that are secreted from glands in order to affect a physical response in the body. How these chemical transmitters are made remains one of life's little mysteries.

To name a few that are directly or indirectly related to the nausea cycle and vomiting we see epinephrine, norepinephrine, acetylcholine, substance P, serotonin, dopamine, and others. The cranial nerves most directly responsible for salivary secretions are the facial, vagus and glossopharyngeal nerves. When stimulated by the central nervous system, messages are sent to a variety of salivary glands (sublingual, submandibular, parotid, etc) telling them to turn on and perform a specific function.

The anatomy, physiology and pharmacology of this subject get significantly more technical and the complexities are beyond the scope of this discussion. For our purposes it is a priority to know that the autonomic nervous system's response during the final stages of the nausea cycle is to heavily stimulate the salivary glands. When this occurs during an extreme autonomic response, specific neurotransmitters are manufactured by and secreted from these glands into your mouth. But what exactly is in that saliva and what is its purpose?

It has been thought for years that the purpose of this heavy salivary flow just prior to vomiting is to protect the teeth and lubricate the esophagus. With the impending release of highly acidic stomach contents during the act of vomiting, it is understandable that the body might secrete this specialized saliva in order to coat and protect the structures of the mouth and throat. This concept has been widely accepted and because it makes perfect sense it has not been questioned or challenged - until now.

The premise and goal of the P-MAV is to consciously sever the link between this specialized saliva and its destination thereby preventing the secreted neurotransmitter from delivering its message. This specialized saliva, from this point forward to be known as vomit saliva or VS, is the key to the entire process. The VS contains the neurotransmitters that are directly and immediately responsible for the process of vomiting to take place. However, without making physical contact with its destination within the gut, these neurotransmitters will not send the signals to the chemoreceptor trigger zone (CTZ) in the brain to induce the vomiting process. It's all about the saliva.

The P-MAV: How is it done?

The procedure for the P-MAV is quite simple. You need to prevent the vomit saliva (VS) from going down your throat and into your stomach by any and all means possible. The easiest way to do this is to not swallow - at all. It is very important to recognize the sudden change in salivary flow from normal saliva (NS) to VS. As soon as this happens, do not swallow. In order to prevent an autonomic reaction, you need to consciously take action at this point before it's too late.

The tricky part, especially for people using the P-MAV for the very first time, is to be aware of these salivary changes when they take place. When you are in the throes of the nausea cycle and especially toward the very end, your mind will start playing tricks on you. You will not be thinking straight and the ONLY thing on your mind will be how miserable you feel. When will it all be over? You almost welcome the vomiting because your previous experiences tell you the nausea will be over after the vomiting. It is very difficult to focus on anything else at this point in time. Do not swallow. This is the number one important message to take away from these instructions.

Just as the VS starts to flow, you will have the urge to swallow and maybe a combination of spitting and swallowing. Resist this urge and don't even spit. When you spit you have a natural tendency to slightly swallow between spitting. The key to the P-MAV is to simply lean forward and let the VS just drip out of your wide open mouth. It would be a good idea to let it drip into the toilet, a sink or a suitable container. Take nice relaxing breaths and just let it all out. At some point it will really start flowing. It will seem as if it's pouring out of your mouth and you will wonder where all of this saliva is coming from. Timing is everything and recognizing the difference between the saliva consistencies will help you determine when to let it flow out.

After you start, the P-MAV takes only about 30 seconds to complete before the VS flow begins to subside. When trying the P-MAV for the first time you may want to start a little earlier than you think is necessary. The VS may catch you by surprise if you wait too long. There is no mistaking the consistency of this saliva as well as the flow rate. You will certainly know when it begins and also when it ends by the sheer volume of saliva that spills from your mouth.

When the heavy flow of saliva stops, the glands that are secreting the VS will stop producing the chemicals that induce vomiting. You will have successfully tricked your body into thinking it has completed the nausea cycle - and essentially it has - only without the contractions, retching, vomiting, foul taste, smell and mess. Miraculously, within seconds you will begin to feel better again with a new lease on life. You will feel so relieved and more importantly feel confident that you have learned a method to avoid the most unpleasant part of the nausea cycle.

Go drink a lot of water to replenish all of the fluids you have lost. Remember, it's a cycle and it may come back around again so be ready and be prepared.

Conclusion

By experimenting with the P-MAV you will quickly become confident in its use and benefit from its advantages when the correct circumstances arise. The P-MAV is specifically intended to avoid vomiting but does not have the capacity to eliminate or avoid the symptoms of nausea or the cause. It is not a cure for sea sickness or morning sickness or any of the other common causes of vomiting. Although it is not a cure, if you can use the P-MAV to eliminate the most uncomfortable part of the illness (the vomiting) then perhaps there will be a significant amount of relief from the overall experience of nausea.

The P-MAV is not fool-proof and may not work 100% of the time. Some ailments which cause instantaneous vomiting without warning or without the typical symptoms associated with the nausea cycle may not respond to the P-MAV. Again, recognizing the appropriate times and situations that the P-MAV will be most beneficial to you is key to its success. When used properly it can result in a quicker recovery from your ailment by eliminating the excess trauma to your system caused by the process of vomiting.

www.ingramcontent.com/pod-product-compliance
Lightning Source LLC
Chambersburg PA
CBHW070923180526
45168CB00005B/2131